M000209257

Satisfying The

BLACK WOMAN

SEXUALLY

Made Simple

By : Dr. Rosie Milligan

Edited By : Pamela Milligan M.D.

Photography By : Roderick Solomon

Design
Layout/Typesetting By : The Fuller Group

Published BY: Professional Business Consultants

©1990 By Dr. Rosie Milligan

ISBN 1-881524-00-0

(REVISED EDITION - MAY 1994)

All rights reserved. No part of this book may be reproduced in whole or in part, in any form or by any means, electronic or mechanical, including photocopying, recording or by any information storage and retrieval system, without permission in writing from the author. Address inquiries to:

Professional Business Consultants
2108 West Manchester, Suite C
Los Angeles, California 90047
(213) 750-3592

SEX

Men have
_____

Lost their Lives for It

Lost their Jobs for It

Left their Wives for It

Left their Children for It

Left School for It

Gone A.W.O.L.
from the Military for It

_____

All for a Little Piece of Real Estate
with Grass Growing on It

This Book Will Teach You How
to Keep Up the Lawn

TABLE OF CONTENTS

Please Note:

The internal and external reproductive organs of the Black woman are the same as women of other ethnic groups. Some of the fears, hang- ups, likes and dislikes about sex may blend in with the women of other races. Therefore, you will find that some issues discussed are not the exclusive feelings of the Black woman. All women share some things in common and there is no getting around it. Nevertheless, my main focus is geared towards the Black woman because of the various social, psychological, and economical factors that have greatly impacted her life and therefore her sexuality.

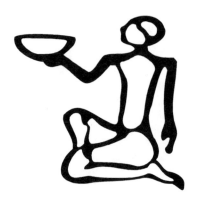

PERSONAL
ACKNOWLEDGEMENTS

I am truly thankful to my friend Barbara Lindsey of Lindsey and Associates for insisting that I write this book. She is a promoter and has been saying for years, "Rosie, you have too much to say, not to say it. I would love to promote you as a speaker but you have got to get some products." Thank you Barbara for pushing excellence.

To my long time friend, Ruby Smith, who has said, "Girl, I see greatness in you." I wish to say thank you for believing in me.

Barbara, Ruby and I have been friends since our high school days. The two of them never allowed me to quit. When I would quit, they would not accept it. They would say, "You have not quit - - you are just resting."

To my friend and business partner, Mary Lee Crump, who has always made "such- to-do" out of everything that I have ever done - - - I thank you for being there for me, emotionally and financially.

I also want to acknowledge my lovely children, Pamela Milligan, M.D., Editor of this book; John Jr., and Cedric, who believes that if I didn't say it, it has no merit nor value.

I want to acknowledge my sisters and brothers who have considered me their mentor, especially my sister, Clara Hunter King, who has shared all of my woes throughout childhood and my young adult life. Thanks, Clara! ... Also, thank you Kenyaka Mamahi, my baby sister, who called everyday to see how far I was from the finishing line on the book. Here it is!

To Armentria Johnson, my godmother, who had all the answers to questions that I could not find during my research - - (she has certainly not been asleep for three scores) -
- I love you.

Special thanks to all those women who participated in the survey. This book is a part of you!

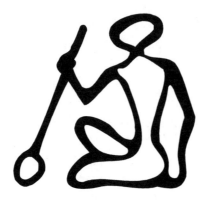

BIOGRAPHY

Dr. Rosie L. Milligan, Registered Nurse, Health Consultant, Author and Ph.D. in Business Administration, has been an achiever most of her life. She has always been involved in a career or business in which she was helping other people accomplish what they want in life. Her motto, "Erase No- - - Step Over Can't- - - and Move Forward with Life," has been a motivating influence to hundreds to whom she has been mentor and role model.

As well as being the mother of three (3) children, Dr. Milligan is also a successful entrepreneur and a national lecturer on male- female relationships, human sexuality, and mental and physical hygiene. Her book, "Satisfying the Black Woman Sexually- - - Made Simple" is rapidly moving toward being a best seller.

Dr. Milligan has taught nursing education and was Director of Nursing for the College of Allied Health Careers and for the Los Angeles Job Corps Center. She assisted in writing the competency- based educational curriculum for Geriatric Nursing for the National Job Corps and holds a life- long teaching credential for the State of California.

As an entrepreneur, the Mississippi native is the owner of PROFESSIONAL BUSINESS CONSULTING SERVICES and hostess of Financial Freedom Forum on Continental Cablevision.

As a successful motivational speaker and trainer, Dr. Milligan has appeared on numerous television and radio shows such as Sally Jessy Raphael in New York; People Are Talking in San Francisco; Maury Povich in New York; A.M. Philadelphia; Evening Exchange in Washington, D.C.; and Stevie Wonder's KJLH Radio Station.

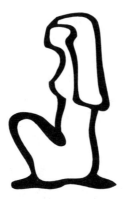

FOREWORD

As the author of nineteen books, a husband for 22 years, and the father of three teenagers, I immediately realized the merit and worth of "Satisfying The Black Woman Sexually". Dr. Rosie Milligan explores a subject which heretofore has been taboo to discuss openly and she does it with humor and a vigor that is simplistically understandable and readable. Moreover, this is a timely topic that needs to be moved out of the barber and beauty shops of the Black community. She has brought the myths out of the closet. She has moved the fears to the forefront so that they can no longer be veiled in ignorance and irrationality.

African American males have long needed this valuable information. Black boys learn sexuality on the streets at an early age often with many misconceptions. This book brings the ebony men and women together in much greater unity than any other book to date.

Since slavery times Black women have been devalued. She is uniquely different from any other woman on the planet and deserves to be treated as such. Dr. Milligan provided men and women with avenues for coming together with warmth, excitement, and fervor, thus alleviating negative stress and uncomfortableness often associated with everyone's deepen inner feelings. Most importantly, she helps us to feel more sure and sensual. She allows us to be more content and makes us want to communicate with each other.

George H. Hill, Ph.D., APR
Hill Cinema/Television Heritage

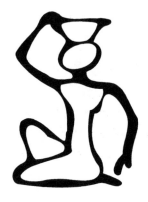

INTRODUCTION

The Black Woman's sexuality is a subject I have wanted to address for a very long time. I hesitated at first because I thought my oldest sister would probably view it as disgracing the family. Secondly, I thought my pastor would probably put me out of the church. Thirdly, I wondered what my children would think or feel. I prayed about it. Then, I called a few friends, like Barbara Lindsey, Mary Crump, Ruby Smith, Jamie Gordon and Kenyaka Mamahi. They were so excited until it made me more excited. As I began to tell them my thoughts, they said, "Hurry and finish! This book is many years late and overdue."

I began to talk to men and women about

my book. The men were just as excited. One male friend asked if he could buy a copy of the handwritten script. He could not wait until it was typed and finished. He needed it right away because he desperately wanted to understand his woman better.

It's kind of funny how most of the men that I have talked with about the book have said, "Oh yes, I have a buddy who really needs this book"...while many women have responded by saying either, "I will surely buy one for my husband," or "I want to read it for myself because I want to know what these men are reading and thinking."

I was telling one of my customers, who is a sixty year old female, about my book. She said, "Oh, that's great. I got married when I was eighteen and I did not enjoy sex until I was thirty- eight." Then she said, "Isn't that ashame?" I replied, "No, it's better late, than never."

I asked my daughter who was a third year medical student to edit my book. She found it to be quite educational. I now see how my book can serve as a love and sex educational guide for my sons. I feel this information can help them with male- female relationships.

I told my sister, Margaret, who talks to my oldest sister, Owen, a lot about writing this book. I also told a church member about the book who is a close friend to my pastor. Whether my oldest sister and my pastor know about this book you are about to read, I do not know. However, I will let you know if I still have an older sister and/or pastor in my next issue.

Chapter

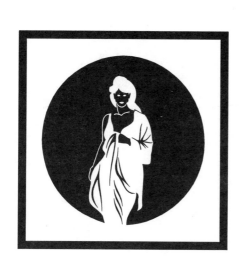

1

The lack of understanding regarding the Black Woman's sexuality and the factors that impact her sexuality are causing serious problems within the Black community. The entire Black community is being jeopardized because of "SEXUALITY CONFUSION."

Haki R. Madhubuti in Black Men Obsolete, Single Dangerous? had the following to say about sexuality.

> "Male and female sexuality has been suppressed by Christian thought. Sexual pleasure in the past has been condemned as a sin, and its suppression has aided men and women in developing new forms of perversion and neurosis. The emergence of rape, pornography and incest (Butler, 1979) is closely related to psycho- sexual problems. The most sought after experience by humans, after eating is sex, and to continuously keep it in the closet will undoubtedly cause serious problems for future generations."

Sex is not everything in a nutshell, however, sex has an effect on everything we do. A couple needs much, much more than sex to bridge and sustain a well-balanced healthy relationship. Sexual activities have a strong influence on the way one thinks and performs in all areas of activity. Ishakamus Barashango in Afrikan Woman the Original Guardian Angel made the following statement regarding sexuality.

> "As evidenced, Puritanical societies where sexual harmony is repressed tend to be more violent and aggressive. Now I am not citing this in a spirit of abject

promiscuity or to emphasize mere biological gratification, but rather as a re-affirmation of ancient Afrikan High Culture societies' general attitudes toward, and genuine concern for, the achievement of a cosmic balance in human sexuality.".

We must understand that cultural differences brings about sexuality differences. Many Black Women want so much to be like the white woman that they defy any notion that they may be different in any fashion.

All women have some things in common and there is no getting around it. Nevertheless, my main focus is geared towards the Black Woman, because of the various social, psycho-logical, and economical factors that have greatly impacted her life and therefore her sexuality. Because of racism, sexism, classism, being the most frequent victim of rape, the woman most frequently left alone to rear her children, and the lowest paid in the employment sector, the Black Woman warrants special sensitivity like:

"STROKING THE MIND, BEFORE STROKING THE BEHIND."

This book is not addressed to the Black man solely. For men of every race, creed and color their greatest fantasy is to make love to a Black Woman. The movies today do such an injustice to the Black Woman. She is so devaluated- - portrayed as a slut or prostitute and called names such as bitch, whore and even more degrading names. This negative impact cause men of other races to continue to want to secretly hang out with the Black Woman.

Dr. Frances Cress Welsign in <u>The Isis Paper</u> states:

> *"For all that we can imagine doing and all that we will do or fail to do is a result of that picture of "self," derived from our total experiences from birth onward. That picture becomes the basis for all our behavioral patterns. Unfortunately, a major part of these self and group images for all too many of us Blacks consists of a brief and inaccurate history."*

The stress imposed on the Black Woman today has taken a toll on her sexuality. The Black Woman wants to satisfy her mate, however she also wants to be satisfied. Any and all frustration absorbs too much energy. Remember sexual activities have a strong influence on the way one thinks and performs in all areas of activity.

Many Black Women suffer depression lasting six months to one year according to leading experts. Some symptoms of depression are excessive sleeping, lack of energy, poor concentration and short attention span. Women taking anti- depressant medications sometime suffer a decline in sex drive and gain weight which adds to the problems already at hand.

According to statistics 46% of Black Women have fibroid tumors far greater than their white counterparts. However, white women often have the fibroid tumors removed surgically while Black Women have hysterectomies. Fibroid tumors cause women to have excessive heavy bleeding during their menstrual cycle, clotting and other menstrual irregularities. The excessive heavy bleeding sometimes causes the woman to suffer a condition called anemia, which causes lack of energy and fatigue. In addition, after having a hysterectomy, many women feel very insecure and less sexually desirable. Also, many men are misinformed about the woman's sexuality after a hysterectomy. Some men think that a woman will not be as good in bed after having a hysterectomy.

It is important that men understand how these dilemmas impact the Black Woman's sexuality. With a clear understanding of these dilemmas men will then be able to embrace the Black Woman with a deeper love and sensitivity.

Chapter

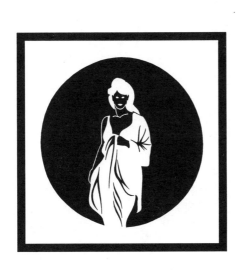

2

My father was frank with me about every issue of life except sex. I remember asking my father (Simon) where babies came from. He said, "The doctor brings them to the house in his little black bag." During those times babies were delivered at home by midwives and doctors. The mother would give the child a name at birth for a midwife to record. Later the child would be given a different name. I have a sister who was given the name Alice at birth, and as such, it is written on her birth certificate. However, we know her as Mary. I once asked my father how her name became changed. He said, "My sister asked your mother how come she did not name that girl after her, and for peace sake, your mother decided that we call her Mary Alice."

I have a cousin that for some unknown reason was always sick. The grown folks often referred to her as the sickly child. However, later in life we all learned that she was never really sick. She just pretended to be ill because she thought the doctor would bring her a baby one day in the little black bag.

Reflecting back on when I was a child, I clearly remember how the grown- ups would come together to discuss certain issues and problems of life. In the majority of cases, you and I both know that those issues involved someone else's business. Therefore, they would often try to talk over our heads using words that they thought were beyond our level of understanding. When a woman or young girl became pregnant, they would discuss it using code words like:

* She is in family way.

* She broke her leg.

* She was stung by the bee.

* She swallowed a watermelon seed.

* She is big.

Most parents never discussed sex or pregnancy in any detailed manner with their children. Their sex education went something like this:

* Gal you keep your dress down, you hear me.

* Don't you come up pregnant.

* Don't you make me shame of you.

* Don't you do nothing nasty with boys.

The one that really puzzled me was "keep you dress down." My sister and I would really laugh at that one. We would always say, "What is she talking about?" (meaning our step- mother). I was always one who wanted answers so I asked, "What do you mean about keeping your dress down?" She said, "You know what I mean and don't ask me a bunch of questions like this, I am going to tell your daddy you are being fast." I said, "Fast, what you mean?" She would answer, "You go and get my belt cause you want to be sassy." I said, "Belt, for what? What did I do?" My sister said, "Shut up girl you do not have to know everything."

When my father came home I reported her. He said, "She got upset cause you were asking about sex." I said, "What is that?" He replied,

"That is something grown folks do." (I was thirteen years old at this time.)

I asked my teacher at school about the matter and she said, "You are getting pretty fast asking these kind of questions." Then, she preceded to tell me all about it. She made me promise not to tell anybody what we had talked about. I became so angry at my step-mother for thinking that I would even consider doing such a nasty thing. My teacher had to tell me every detail because I would not stop at incomplete answers. Our conversation went like this:

Me: How do you do sex?

Teacher:
The woman lies down and opens her legs, the man lies on top after putting his thang into her 'kitty cat".

Me: His 'thang', what is that?

Teacher:
The thing between his legs that he pees out of.

Me: Oh that is nasty. And what is a kitty cat ?

Teacher:
A 'Kitty Cat' is the thing between a womans's legs where she pees from.

Me: Oh that is nasty.

Teacher:
It is nasty only when girls do it. It is O.K. for grown married people. You see, that is how you got here. That is how your mother got pregnant.

Me: She got pregnant, what is that?

Teacher:
Pregnancy is when the man does the sex thing with a woman and a baby grows inside her stomach.

Me:
You mean I was inside my mother's stomach? How did I get in there and how did I get out?

At this point, she explained in detail and step- by- step until I understood. Then she said to me, "You are a nosey little something. You will probably be a scientist."

I thought to myself, if my parents wanted to whip me for just talking about sex, then they would surely kill me if I did it.

I began to teach sex education to my classmates- - the little bit I had learned from my teacher. I had them to swear they would never tell the lessons they had learned. I taught them the proper names for the male and female sex organs. Below is a list of names we called the vagina:

* Kitty Cat	* Poontang	* Cooche
* Pussy	* Cock	* Pocket book
* The Beaver	* Trim	* Booty
* Snatch		

Below is a list of names we called the penis:

* Thang	* Pee Pee	* Dick

* Rod   * Dingerling   * Peter

* Johnson

All the kids thought I was so smart. In addition to being an `A' student, my fellow classmates saw me as also having street smarts, or shall I say road smarts because we did not know the term "street." We had roads.

When I was fifteen, I was captain of the high school basketball team. I was very popular with the boys. I developed friendships with mostly boys; because I wanted to know more about them. I also hung with my male cousins a lot. I have always loved being around men. I guess it is because I saw them as being an extension of my father who was the most beautiful man in the world. I spent most of my time with my father.

I would often go out on the field to practice basketball while the boys were practicing. However, sometimes the boys got angry. I had to plead with the coach to let me stay. I convinced him that playing was something I loved more than life itself. He would say to the boy's team, "Leave her alone, she is not hurting a thing." When they would stop for breaks, they would sometimes talk vulgar to make me want to leave. Nevertheless, I stayed right there. I would laugh with them. Despite this, I was loved by the boys and the girls alike because I was good at keeping the secrets of both sexes.

I have always liked hanging out with people from whom I could learn. I would ask questions until I was satisfied with the answers.

I am so happy that sex education is taught

at an early age in school nowadays. I am glad it is taught in a positive fashion. However, it can be taken to the extreme when taught by teachers who lack true morals.

I have talked with many Black Women who freely shared with me the negative information that was taught to them in the early years. This misinformation severely impacted their sex lives, often in a detrimental fashion. When a woman has been programmed that sex is something bad and nasty, it is kind of hard to make it turn into something good and beautiful just because she has marched down an aisle and stood before a preacher.

In retrospect, I feel that parents did not object to their daughters having sex, but objected to them getting pregnant. I often wondered if those parents were absolutely sure that their daughters would not get pregnant, would they have viewed sex in a different manner. Would they have painted a more warm and beautiful picture about sex, instead of painting a picture of a man that would make a woman flee from him? For example, parents often used old familiar quotes and scare tactics such as:

> *A man will sleep around with you and when he is ready for a wife he will take a virgin.*
> *No man wants a ready-made family, when he is perfectly capable of making his own.*
> *Why buy the cow, if you can have the milk for free.*

You may think this is old, outdated information, but it is not. This type of teaching is still going on and has been passed on for generations. Some of us have broken free from the chains of guilt, shame and fear taught to us about our sexuality and sexual nature. Some of us have not and some of us never will.

Interestingly, I am by no means saying that these problems, teachings and behaviors are common only in the Black family. I conducted a survey on other ethnic groups regarding their cultural perspective and behaviors in relation to pre- marital sex, ready- made families, pregnancy without marriage, sickness and health, old wise sayings, superstitions, etc. I have spent a lot of time with many different ethnic groups as a nurse, nursing instructor and as a friend. In this book, however, I am only addressing the sexuality and highest sexual fulfillment of the Black Woman.

This book is not addressed to the Black Man solely. We know that men of every creed and color desire the forbidden fruit, *the Black Woman*. Therefore, this book is to any and every man who has chosen the Royal Queen to be a co-partner in ruling his dynasty. This book will help you enjoy the finest experience life has to offer on this earth. As quoted by Dr. Yosef A. A. Ben-Joshannan:

"Heaven is between a Black Woman's legs."

I would like to modify his statement by saying:

"Heaven on Earth is between a Black Woman's legs."

I do believe that there is a Heaven that God has prepared for prepared people.

Chapter

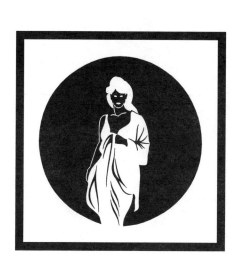

3

The Black Woman Before Slavery

According to studies, the majority of Black people brought to America came from West African societies. It was during the late seventeenth, eighteenth, and early nineteenth centuries that Black African women were brought to America.

The Black Woman played roles that were most vital to the survival of her people. Her most important function was motherhood. She was highly visible in the economic marketplace, controlling certain industries such as: sewing and selling cloth, pottery, trading and selling of goods of various kinds. Because the Black Woman held a high economic position, many became independently wealthy. She also had the responsibility of raising food for her family by planting crops and attending to them.

The Black Woman took care of her children and prepared meals for her husband. She had less physical obligations with her husband because, more than likely, he had more than one wife.

The Black Woman's role as a mother took priority over her husband and the marketplace. When she became pregnant she would leave her husband's house and go to her father's house. She stayed there until her baby was weaned usually for approximately 3 years. The same routine was repeated with each pregnancy. One can see clearly that the Black Woman lived as an independent woman with her children. The children went everywhere with the mother, tied to her back. The children were very close to their mothers. The strongest bond in slavery was that between mother and child.

The Black Woman felt very good about herself. There was no doubt regarding her being the essence of femininity and beauty. There was no thought or idea about measuring up to some one else's standard of beauty. The African Woman was the standard by which beauty was measured.

Many loving relationships have been ruined between the Black Woman and her man because of a lack of knowledge about the Black Woman's history.

By now I am sure you are wondering when is Dr. Milligan going to get to the part on sexuality. Well, in all actuality, I have been talking about it for a while. Now, if you do not agree with me, just try to be romantic or to make love to a Black woman when she does not know the whereabouts of her child.

Chapter

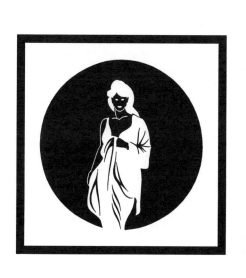

4

The Effects of Slavery on
The Black Woman's Sexuality

Did you know that the Black Woman did not come to America on an Airplane? She was thrown on the same slave ship as the Black man. The Black Woman was exploited as a laborer in the fields. The Black Woman was also exploited as a breeder, a domestic household worker, and as a sex object for the white man. The Black Woman was also branded with a hot iron and was beaten severely when she cried during the process. She was forced to take off her clothing so she could be beaten on all parts of her body. The Black woman was forced to walk around naked as a constant reminder of her sexual vulnerability.

Bell Hooks in her book, AIN'T A WOMAN, had the following to say regarding the Black Woman's slave experience.

> African females received the brunt of this mass brutalization and terrorization not only because they could be victimized via their sexuality but also because they were more likely to work intimately with the white family than the black male. Since the slaver regarded the black woman as a marketable cook, wet nurse, and housekeeper, it was crucial that she be so thoroughly terrorized that she would submit passively to the will of the white master, mistress, and their children. In order to make his product saleable, the slaver had to ensure that no resistant black female servant would poison a family, kill children, set fire to the house, or resist in any way.

The Black Woman was stripped of her dignity on every level. She was raped and beaten by white men and Black men alike. She was often used by the white man for various selfish motives in which she had no choice and no rights, such as:

> * *To increase the family size for the sole purpose of producing new slave hands.*

> * *To take care of their children's physical and emotional needs. (They were amazed at how the Black Woman was able to modify their spoiled rotten children's behavior in a positive way by giving them love. The white children could feel the love that radiated from the Black Woman. This is the reason they would run up to hug her when their parents were out of their sight, in spite of the low- down evil talk about Blacks they had heard from their parents and family members during open conversations.)*

> * *To help work the cotton fields.*

> * *To give him an earthly- heavenly experience when between her legs.*

I once had a conversation with an old White man in Mississippi who I knew through my father because they were both farm owners. I remember asking him specifically whether or not it was pure hatred for the Black Woman that made white men rape her. I was shocked and astounded to find out through his response that it was not pure hatred, but pure lust for the Black Woman's beautiful body that led to such a violent act. He went on to describe how beautifully rounded the shape of her butt was and how much pleasure and excitement he got from riding by in his truck watching the Black women bent over working in the fields. Then he talked about how large their breasts were as they stood at attention like a soldier in the army. As I stood listening, I was totally amazed and overwhelmed as I thought- - "Wow! All this time I thought they hated the very sight of the Black Woman, but it was just the opposite."

In the fundamentalist Christian teaching, woman was viewed as an evil sexual temptress. A white woman desiring sex was seen as a degraded and immoral human being. The white woman who suppressed her sexual feelings was looked upon as a goddess, innocent, pure and holy rather than a worldly person. I like the way Bell Hooks described the white woman's dilemma:

> "Once the white female was mythologized as pure and virtuous, a symbolic Virgin Mary, white men could see her as exempt from negative sexist stereotypes of the female. The price she had to pay was the suppression of natural sexual impulses. Given the strains of endless pregnancies and the hardships of childbirth, it is understandable that 19th- century white women felt no great attachment to their sexuality and gladly accepted the new, glorified desexualized identity white men imposed upon them."

Black Women were viewed as sexually promiscuous savages. Bell Hooks had the following to say about this subject matter:

> Since women were designated as the orig-
> inator of sexual sin, the Black women were
> naturally seen as the embodiment of female
> evil and sexual lust. They were labeled
> Jezebels and sexual temptresses and
> accused of leading white men away from
> spiritual purity into sin. One white
> politician urged that the blacks be sent back
> to Africa so that white men would not for-
> nicate and commit adultery. His words
> were "remove this temptation from us."

Many white men had their very first (and
best) sexual encounters with a Black woman so
that they could keep their women pure and
unspoiled until marriage. They raped the young
black female usually by the age of thirteen and
older. The white men found much, much
pleasure in having sex with the Black Woman.
He acquired an addiction for her body sexually
and even after entering into marriage, he con-
tinued to sneak out of his house in the late hours
of the night to find pleasure by having sex with
the Black Woman.

Whenever the white man was caught in the
act of raping a Black woman, the Black woman
was severely beaten and given harsh punishment
by the white woman.

White women were the most cruel towards
the Black Woman during slavery because she
envied the body that the White man lusted for
day and night. When the Black Woman gave
birth to a mixed baby, the White women knew
that some White woman's husband was the
father. The white woman always tried to make

the Black Woman feel ugly, less than a woman, and less than a human being.

Some Black Women today are still ashamed of their bodies if they have a few extra pounds here and there, especially, if they are well endowed in the hip, thigh and breast areas.

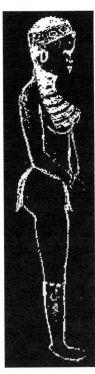
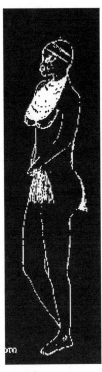
The Black Woman is a very shapely, sensuous woman. She is often so obsessed with the European standard of beauty of being five feet six, size six dress, size seven shoe, waist of 22 inches, small breasts, thin lips, green and blue eyes, etc. that she sometimes forgets the unique beauty of the African woman. The Black Woman's perfect breasts, broad hips and her beautiful thick lips, are envied all around the world.

As a result of the impact of slavery, many Black Women today have not learned to appreciate their physical differences and therefore have not learned to express their sexuality fully.

Many Black Women spend countless hours trying to work off their cushion (healthy buttocks). They do not realize that men are experiencing much pleasure as a result of her well endowed behind (cushion).

Picture a typical Black woman lying in bed on her back. Visualize her body, her rounded well endowed behind places her body in a exciting position. Visualize her body lying on her side. Visualize her body standing in an erect position. The Black Woman's body is sensuous from any angle East, West, North and South. Now picture a woman with a flat behind lying in bed in the same position. Men find themselves having to place their hands under her buttocks to elevate her buttocks in a position that is a natural position for a typical Black woman.

A man making love to a woman with well endowed buttocks can find other uses for his hands to bring about even more pleasure. Most Black Women are not aware that they have been blessed with a built in comfortable rocking chair (cushion).

Chapter

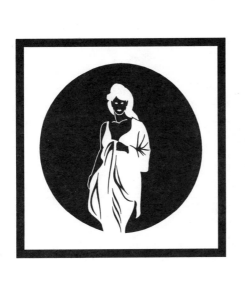

5

The Kind of Man A Black Woman Wants

The Black Woman wants a man who is sensitive to her past, present and future. One who is caring, gentle, thoughtful and respectful.

Sensitive .... *Enough to measure the Black Woman with the right meter stick. Beginning at the point where she entered the race.*

Caring .... *Enough to help her cross over the barriers in her past and present life's experiences that prohibit the enjoyment and gratification of a loving relationship.*

Enough to ensure total sexual satisfaction for his Black woman.

Gentle .... *Enough to caress with tenderness.*

Enough not to provoke pain during intercourse.

Enough to assist in putting on coats and opening and closing doors.

Thoughtful ..... *Enough to remember birthdays, anniversaries, etc.*

Enough to give a pleasant surprise every now and then.

Enough to help do the housework.

* Knowing that in todays's family many women are in the work place because two incomes are needed.

Enough to make life exciting and exhilarating by:

* Preparing the bath water.
* Laying out a favorite outfit he likes to see his woman wear.

* Sending flowers on a non special occasion - - - just because I love you. I appreciate you. You are my woman.

Enough to say thank you for things such as:

* A Compliment.
* A special meal.
* A romantic evening.
* A good sexual surprise

Respectful ..... *Enough to call on the telephone when coming home at an unusual time.*

Enough to respect a difference of opinion on issues.

If by now you are questioning what does all of this have to do with sex, my answer to this question would be, "What does baking powder have to do with a cake? What does yeast have to do with bread? It makes it rise."

If you think that what I have been talking about has nothing to do with sex, then I challenge you to try all of the above suggestions and you will see that you will be the world's most sexually satisfied man. If you choose not to take heed, then you go right ahead and I will tell your story in my next volume.

Chapter

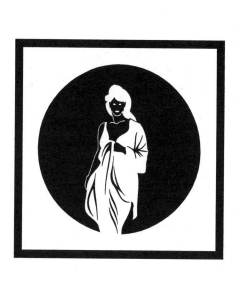

6

W hat the Black Woman wants as a whole from her man or lover is openness and honesty, respect, sensitivity, and fairness. She would like the freedom of not being expected or pressured to engage in every sexual practice invented if it is outside her comfort zone or conflicts with her inner beliefs. The Black Woman likes to know that she is winning during sexual intercourse. She likes a man who is sensitive enough to communicate his likes and dislikes about sex and welcomes her likes and dislikes. A man whose masculinity is not threatened when she guides him into positions and areas that she finds more fulfilling by expressing or stating phases such as:

> *Come up a little higher*
> *Move more to the left*
> *Move more to the right*
> *Move down a little lower*
> *Move a little slower*
> *Let us try a new routine*
> *Wait until it gets harder*

A Black woman's sexual experiences, social setting of which she was reared, physical capabilities, religious background and up bringing, all have a strong impact and influence on how she genuinely feels about sex, how much she enjoys sex, and her willingness to explore various positions and exotic practices during sex. This is the main reason why the Black Woman's history was expounded on in the previous chapters, so that you would have a better insight of the present nature of the Black Woman- - - as a reflection of her past. To understand the present condition of any sex or race, the past condition or history must be examined and understood If a Black Woman has a personal history or family history of rape, she certainly will not enjoy any act that makes her feel helpless, controlled or violated, like the whip and chain approach when the woman is slapped, scratched or abused on any parts of her boy.

The Black Woman does not like to be called names such as bitch or whore while making love. She does not find such sexual practice to be romantic or sexually fulfilling. All men must realize that the Black Woman is from a different experience. She has a background and history of her own that is far different from women of other ethnic groups. Nevertheless, there are also differences between Black Women in their likes and dislikes about sex, and therefore these things should be communicated between sexual partners.

While some Black Women may have no sexual limitations or inhibitions, other Black Women may find certain request asked of them by their lovers to be demeaning and degrading.

There is one sexual factor that I believe all women have in common and this is the desire to reach the highest level of sexual fulfillment- - - Orgasm.

I asked a friend one day why did he take drugs. He told me that drugs made him feel like he was floating in another world that was free of care with a one way ticket. Later I asked him about how long that feeling lasted. He said, less than a minute. Then, I responded, "Wow, that sounds like an orgasm to me." We laughed for awhile about my remark and then he admitted that he was shocked that I, Ms. Professional Woman, would say this. I then reminded him that women- - - short, tall, big, or small, professional, nonprofessional, skilled, unskilled, Christian and non- Christians- - - all have basic needs for sexual fulfillment.

It is important that one understands the female sexual response cycle in order to understand sexual phases. I like the way the female sexual response cycle is explained in the book entitled, <u>Understanding Human Behavior In Health and Illness</u>, Third Edition, edited by Richard C. Simons, M.D.

(see chart on next page)

The Female Sexual Response Cycle

I. EXCITEMENT
(several minutes to hours)

No change

Nipple erection, Venous congestion
Areolar enlargement

II. PLATEAU
(30 seconds to 3 minutes)

Sexual flush: Inconstant may
appear on face, neck, breast
abdomen, or thigh, may
resemble measles rash

Venous pattern prominent. Size
may increase 1/4 over resting state

Areolae enlarges and impinges on
nipples so they seem to disappear

III. ORGASMIC
(3 to 15 seconds)

No change

No change

IV. RESOLUTION
(10 to 15 min., if no orgasm $1/2$ to 1 day)

Flush disappears in reverse
order

Return to normal

CLITORIS	UTERUS
Glans: Diameter increased Shaft: Variable increase in diameter Elongation occurs in 10% of subjects	Ascends into false pelvis in phase I
Retraction: Shaft withdraws deep into swollen prepuce	Contractions: Strong sustained contractions begin late in Phase II
No change (shaft movement continue throughout if thrusting is maintained)	Contractions strong throughout orgasm. Strongest with pregnancy and masturbation
Shaft returns to normal position in 5 - 10 secs., full detumescence in 5 - 10 min.	Slowly returns to normal position

A woman wants her man to know when she is ready for intercourse. Oftentimes, a man is ready even before his woman takes off her clothes. Many men need to understand that their readiness is not a ready signal for their women. Men, please repeat the above sentence ten times.

An erection for a man is equivalent to lubrication for a woman. The male erection and female lubrication both signify readiness for intercourse. A man cannot have intercourse if he does not have an erection, but a woman does not have to lubricate in order to have intercourse. It may be uncomfortable if she does not lubricate, but there are ways around that. Saliva or a lubricator may be used.

A woman wants a man who is in tune and in touch with her body language.

Touching for pleasure is so very important because it gives the man an opportunity to tune into his woman's body talk. While touching for pleasure, observe her sexual response. When she is in the excitement phase notice:

- *Her breathing*
- *Her skin color*
- *Her firm grip as she holds you*
- *Her eyes*
- *Her body movements*
- *The sound she makes as you touch and stroke her body*
- *How she calls your name*
- *Her breast, how the nipples become erect*

The nipple erection is due to contraction of muscle fiber and not because of increased blood flow, which is responsible for many of the other changes noted in the body during sexual excitement.

Men, I say unto you, by the power vested in me, that by the above, you should know when your woman is ready for you. Forget what men have taught you. Trust me, when your woman is "Ripe Ready." She will guide your penis in the direction that it should go. Lose control - - - lay aside your ego at this time and allow your woman to take you where she wants you to go. I realize that you feel that it is your job to be in the driver's seat; however, allow your woman to park the car in the garage. You just go for the ride and enjoy your heavenly experience.

Some men think that every time they feel wetness inside the vagina the woman has had an orgasm. However, this is not always the case. Often the secretions felt are due to the friction and stimulation which occur during foreplay or after the penis has entered the vagina.

When a woman is experiencing an orgasm, both partners can actually feel the muscles of the uterus contracting. There is also a change in her breathing rate, it will increase according to the intensity of her pleasure. The woman's eyes are either closed or opened with an upward fixed stare, or they open and close at the rhythm of her breathing. Sometimes her body becomes rigid and is then followed by a state of softness and relaxation. At other moments her body may undergo an uncontrollable tremble or jerkily movement. Some women bodies slip into such a deep state of relaxation they fall asleep. While other women feel a surge of energy that gives them an overwhelming desire to experience a second burst of pleasure.

Anything short of the description above has been a fun and enjoyable evening without an orgasm. This does not mean that a woman did not enjoy having sex because she did not have an orgasm. Some women look forward to foreplay only with her man and would be pleased if he went no further. Some women dislike foreplay and would like to get right to the physical activity. In order to make each sexual experience more fulfilling you must find out what your partner likes. Therefore, it would be wise to discuss the do's and dont's list. Think of what could happen if your woman is about to have an orgasm and you touched one of the don't spots. Remember, messing up a woman's chance for an orgasm is an unforgivable sin.

You should find out what your woman would like for you to do when she is experiencing an orgasm. She might want you to hold still or stop all movements. Some men tend to want to get real busy during that time. I guess they feel that since they brought you to the mountain top they want to push you over it. Sometimes certain movements decrease the intensity of an orgasm.

An orgasm is a wonderful experience; however, a woman can enjoy sex and live a happy life without it. Most women never knew they had not been having an orgasm until they finally had one. It may be to her advantage to continue enjoying her man without an orgasm because once she experiences it, she will want it every time. She may even become frustrated without it, because now she knows what she is missing.

It is not the sole responsibility of the man to bring his woman to ecstasy. The woman is equally responsible for her own sexual gratification. A woman is capable of having more orgasms repetively by herself through masturbation than any man can cause her to have. Therefore, when it comes to the "Big O" (orgasm), a man is a luxury and not a necessity.

It is a good idea for sexual partners to explore each other's body and encourage each other to explore his or her body alone. It should become a joint venture to assure the highest possible sexual gratification for both partners. Sexual research has shown that women who use self- stimulation become orgasmic.

The book entitled The Sensuous Woman by "J" so plainly gives a message to the woman.

> "When you have educated your body to the point where it can reel off several orgasms at your command, you will be able to guide him when making love to positions that give you the maximum sensation. After all, if you do not know what sets your body off sensually, how can you expect him to know? Every woman is different, and he's not clairvoyant.

If your woman suffers hang- ups in this area, then it is your responsibility to help her cross those barriers in order that the two of you can have an enjoyable and healthy relationship. Many times the touching experience for partners are geared toward producing erotic feelings with sexual intercourse as the objective. I like the way Adele P. Kennedy and Susan Dean, Ph.D. add flavor to the art of touching in their book Touching for Pleasure.

> "Foreplay is usually thought of as a prelude to intercourse frequently becoming only a quick route to orgasm. If you can think of foreplay in a new way, as a total experience of its own, you will have added something of value to your pleasuring repertoire."

Men have a greater challenge than women when it comes to physical sex. The man has to focus on getting an erection and keeping the erection until his partner is satisfied. That can become a big challenge especially when the woman takes no responsibility for her own desired results. A man becomes embarrassed when he cannot get an erection. He is also embarrassed when he cannot keep an erection. Let me explain my theory for this dilemma.

The EGO Versus PENIS Syndrome. With this syndrome, a man is overly anxious not to have a floppy penis before he arrives at home base. Therefore, during foreplay, the minute he feels a good erection, he is ready to put it into the vagina no matter what, because he is unsure as to how long the erection will last. He is obsessed with the idea that he must have an orgasm. He will not ask his partner if she is ready for him. In fact, he cannot bring himself to care at this point about what she is feeling. He is only concerned about his ego and erected penis at this time. Therefore, he tries to rush his woman into what he is feeling. He may begin by saying words such as, "Come on Baby. Come with me." In order to save his ego when his woman cannot make it with him, she fakes it. This syndrome is what has brought about the old saying,

"BIP BAM AND THANK YOU MA'AM."

Bob Schwartz, in his book, The One Hour Orgasm states:

> "...another problem is that we, as men, have very seldom been told the truth about our performance with women... until we marry one of them. Men that are the most handsome, rich, or popular, suffer the most from being lied to about how well they perform.
>
> Handsome, rich, and popular men are the most sought after by women. A smart woman does not want to run a man off by stepping on his ego, and the area that is the most important and sensitive to a man is his performance, especially in bed."

We cannot over emphasize the importance of sexuality and the necessity of an orgiastic experience. It is believed that an orgasm does relieve stress and tension very effectively. A woman may exhibit bizarre behavior patterns as a result of not being able to discharge accumulated energy charges.

The following is a description of the orgasmic experience as stated by Dr. William Reich, a psychiatrist, in the book The Holistic Health Handbook, compiled by The Berkeley Holistic Health Center.

"In describing the ideal orgastic experience, which culminates in a total release of sexual energy, Reich identified four distinct and necessary states of energetic process. They are (1) tension, (2) charge, (3) discharge, and (4) relaxation. Together these stages make up what is called the "orgasm cycle.

If this cycle is blocked or incomplete at any point in its progression, the person will not experience a full orgasm, and the energetic charge will continue to animate the bodymind, becoming stored in the neuromuscular system. Unreleased charge will continue to accumulate in this way, creating even more physical and emotional stress and conflict. The sexually potent individual, on the other hand, can move fluidly through the four stages of the orgasm cycle, and can therefore not only give in to the vegetative current of the sexual experience, but also benefit from the psychosomatic cleansing effects of all the full orgiastic release."

I truly hope that you understand how important it is to make a sexual experience a totally gratifying encounter.

A woman does not like for her man to continue asking her did she come. It places the non-assertive woman in an awful position. She is forced to lie in order to spare her man's ego; if she is a woman who seeks to please rather than be pleased. After being dishonest about the issue, she is left frustrated because she is not assertive enough to ask for what she needs from her man so that she may reach her climax with his assistance.

We must understand that women do not come every time they have sex, particularly with only penile thrusting, whether deep or shallow stroking. Some women will not come every time no matter what is done. it is important that men are aware of the female sexual response cycle. This knowledge will help men increase their woman's chance of experiencing an orgasm because he will know when she is ready for intercourse.

When a woman does not come during intercourse, it does not mean that that the man has failed. Neither does it mean that she did not enjoy having the man make love to her; providing that he did make love to her.

Let's take a look at the difference in making love and having sex. You are having sex when there is no foreplay and no afterplay. This type of sex provokes double agony for the woman, especially when a man is a premature ejaculator. (A premature ejaculator is a man who orgasms too soon every time or almost every time he makes love.) A premature ejaculator who is not open to oral sex should equip himself with knowledge and proper usage of sexual toys.

I discovered during my research that some men are intimidated by sexual toys. One reason is that men worry as much about the size of their penis as women do about the their breast size. Sexual toys should be viewed as a sexual pleasure enhancer and not a penis replacement or substitute. Sexual toys are not an enemy to a man. They can be a man's friend. Remember, sexual toys are to sex as salt and pepper is to a steak. Does salt and pepper replace the steak?

When a man has been grumpy and argumentative all day, with his lips poked out, and has not uttered one kind word to his woman, then comes to bed and engages in intercourse as though his attitude has been superb, this is not making love. This is having sex.

When a man sits down and read the newspaper and watches television without volunteering to assist his woman in any fashion while she cooks, does the dishes, helps the children with schoolwork, etc.; and he observes his wife getting in bed for the night but continues to watch T.V. until his story ends, then gets in bed and wakes his woman to satisfy his sexual needs, this is *having* sex.

Lovemaking should not be routine with a schedule cemented in stone; however, it should be conducive to both partner's enjoyment and fulfillment. Dr. Joyce Brothers had the following to say:

> *"Something as simple as changing your sex timetable might make all the difference in the world in the performance of the man in your life. You can take advantage of the low production of the anti-sex hormones and of the high production of testosterone by shifting your lovemaking to the morning hours when male hormone levels are at their peak."*

Making love is when a man takes the time to provide all the foreplay necessary to prepare his woman for a satisfying sexual experience.

There is much dialogue regarding foreplay

and afterplay. I discovered during my research that many women feel that they are not receiving enough foreplay and most of the time, no afterplay.

The assumption is that all men know how to provide adequate foreplay and afterplay; and that all men understand the importance of foreplay and afterplay. I am compelled to describe foreplay because of the response I received during my research survey.

While conducting a workshop on sexual empowerment, I taught lessons on masturbation and the usage of vibrators. A female attendee was very excited and likewise shared the information with her male friend. Her male friend said to her, "The day you purchase a vibrator, count me out of your life because I have a real thing, so why do you need a substitute." Some men think that women use vibrators only for vaginal penetration and thrusting. Many women use vibrators because they prefer it rather than their hands for stimulating the clitoris. I like what Berni Zilbergeld, Ph.D. had to say about the subject:

> *"The clitoris is, for most women, the site of their most intense pleasure. When women masturbate, they typically do so by rubbing on or near the clitoris. (The clitoris is so sensitive in many women that they prefer stimulation to the right or left of it rather than actually on it.) Rarely do they insert anything into the vagina. By now it is widely accepted that clitoral stimulation is what lead to orgasm in most women."*

Having sex is when a man communicates his likes and dislikes but does not solicit the likes and dislikes of his woman. Having sex is when a man orgasms and then falls asleep on top of his woman or just rolls over in bed and goes to sleep. To feel sleepy is natural, however, one does not have to give in to this feeling.

Dr. Joyce Brothers explains this dilemma in her book, <u>What Every Woman Should Know About Men</u>:

> *"During lovemaking, a chemical is released that makes a man feel overpoweringly sleepy- - sleepy, mind you. Not tired. he does not have to give in to the feeling. If he will just make an effort to talk to you, to whisper all those sweet nothings you like to hear, for thirty to forty- five seconds after lovemaking, the urge to sleep will disappear. If he is not aware of this, I suggest that you tell him in your own self- interest. Afterplay is as delicious in its own way as foreplay."*

Foreplay is....whispering sweet things in the ears , lip kissing, tongues kissing, hugging, rubbing, massaging the body, kissing the face, kissing the neck, kissing, the earlobes, kissing the nipples, stroking the body with the tongue, lightly inserting fingers into the vagina and continuing with light gentle thrusting strokes, massaging the clitoris.

A more in depth discussion on foreplay is discussed in Chapter Eleven, "The Recipe for Sexual Fulfillment."

Afterplay is hugging ... holding ... kissing ... and whispering sweet words in the ear after reaching a climax. Some men do not perform after-play for fear that their woman will become sexually aroused again and demand another round. some men, especially men over forty are not capable of obtaining a second erection within an hour and sometimes days. It is not necessary for a man to obtain a second erection in order to give his woman a second burst of pleasure. if a man follows the suggestions mentioned in describing foreplay; his woman could come many more times. Many women describe their second climax as being more intense than the first one.

Making love is when a man expresses his sexual likes and dislikes and is not threatened when a woman expresses her likes and dislikes. In fact, he solicits them.

Making love is when a man recognizes the fact that women are different. Therefore, he searches for his woman's erogenous zones.

Bernie Zilbergeld, Ph.D., in his book, The New Male Sexuality, had the following to say:

> "Although I've already made a number of statements about what is and is not likely to lead to orgasm, I should add a qualification. Erogenous zones and orgasms vary from woman to woman. While a significant minority of women do not find breast stimulation arousing, there are some who can orgasm solely from such stimulation. There is also a small number who can orgasm solely by means of fantasy."

Making love is when a man provides after-play for his woman, recognizing that many times he is the only one that has experienced an orgasm. Concerning this, Zilbergeld had the following to say:

> "The physical changes that occur with orgasm also occur without it, in both women and men, but more slowly. Not orgasming is not a tragedy for either sex. Emotionally, however, it can be something else, depending on the woman's perceptions. If she feels good about the relationship and believes her partner is interested in her satisfaction, it's usually no big deal if she doesn't have an orgasm today. On the other hand, if she feels that the man cares only about his own satisfaction and isn't willing to do anything for her, there will be problems."

Making love is when a man realizes that sex does not begin in the bedroom. Sex is a part of the daily activities and chores from sun up to sun down.

Do not read me wrong. A little quickie is alright for both the man and woman alike, however, if a quickie is all one wants and needs at the time, it should be clearly communicated to his/her partner. After all, who wants to prepare for a long trip when in reality you are only taking them around the corner.

I cannot conclude this chapter without discussing male impotency and premature ejaculation, since it is so prevalent today. What does the Black Woman want from her man in bed? She wants, she needs and she expects, sexual gratification. As long as a man's hands are intact, no matter what else is going on or taking place, his woman should never be sexually frustrated.

I will conclude this chapter with a discussion on male impotency and premature ejaculation; their causes and effects on sexuality in regards to satisfying the Black Woman sexually.

MALE IMPOTENCY. Impotence is the failure to achieve an erection, ejaculation, or both. men who experience sexual dysfunction express the following complaints: loss of sexual desire, not being able to obtain or maintain an erection, ejaculatory failure, premature ejaculation and the inability to achieve orgasm.

In the past, impotence was considered to be 90 percent in a man's head. Because of ignorance, many men today do not seek medical help for impotency. It is now believed that the majority of impotent men have a component of underlying organic disease. Some common causes of erectile impotence and lack of sexual desire in men are boredom, resentment, anger, grief, anxiety, depression, diabetes, and prescription drugs such as anti- hypertensives (used for treating high blood pressure), anti- depressants (used for treating depression and anxiety), anti- cholinergic (used for treating ulcers), and drugs of habituation or addiction such as alcohol, methadone, heroin, cocaine, and marijuana. Some experts believe that we are seeing more impotence in men today because the modern day woman is demanding equal joy in sex. Women are educated consumers regarding sex. More is being written about sex and women are speaking out on national television talk shows, etc. Women are now more sexually aggressive and feel entitled to sexual satisfaction and demand it. This assertiveness of the modern day female has created performance anxiety among men.

Many men entering into a sexual experience are afraid that they may not meet the woman's expectations. Those anxieties can cause problems such as impotence. The Big "O" is the talk of the time; therefore, men are feeling pressured to guarantee women an orgasmic experience every times during sexual intercourse.

It is important for a male to have a thorough physical examination if he has demonstrated little or no interest in sex for a long period of time. A man's impotence is said to be psychological if he can get an erection by masturbating or looking at pornography, has early morning erections, and if he can have an erection with another woman.

Intermittent impotence has been found to be caused by an endocrine imbalance. Endocrine problems are very sneaky. Their only symptom may be that of impotence. A man experiencing impotence should ask his doctor to check his testosterone level. Testosterone is a male hormone. a man has an erection when blood floods through the penile arteries into the blood vessels in the penis. This rush of blood is triggered by the nervous system, which gets its signal from the sex hormones.

Impotence can be a symptom of a number of life- threatening diseases. It is one of the symptoms of diabetes. Diabetes can cause impaired circulation; remember a good erection is a good blood flow to the penis. Diabetes may damage or destroy the nerves that trigger the rush of blood to the penis. According to research, more than three hundred thousand men a year are diagnosed with diabetes. More than half of them are or may be impotent. Diabetic- caused impotence is usually not curable.

PREMATURE EJACULATION. This disorder seldom has an organic cause. It is usually related to anxiety in the sexual situation, unreasonable expectations about performance, or an emotional disorder. Black men are burdened down with sexual stereotyping regarding their sexuality. They have been labeled as "Mandingo," "Long John Silver" and Eveready Battery." The Black man takes these burdens to the bedroom. Therefore, he is pressured more to be an excellent performer in bed.

The size of the penis provokes much anxiety for the male. Men are more concerned about the length of their penis. The average penis is three to four inches long and grows to six inches or so when erected. Most men do not know that the circumference of the penis is more important when it comes to a woman's pleasure. The thicker the penis, the more it will stimulate the clitoris and the lower third of the vagina during intercourse, as this is from where the great sensations come.

It is believed that more men suffer from premature ejaculation than from impotence. A premature ejaculator may ejaculate as soon as his penis enters the vagina. Some even start on the way in. All men have experienced premature ejaculation at one time or another. It happens to young men engaging in sexual intercourse for the first time almost always. Men with experience come too soon sometimes because of intense excitement, anxiety or fatigue.

The man who is considered a true premature ejaculator is the man who comes too soon every time or almost every time he makes love. This is a very humiliating, devastating and embarrassing situation for a man.

Some men are considerate, thoughtful and loving enough to compensate for this weakness by bringing their partner to orgasm before they become aroused or at least before entering the vagina. Some men just stop having intercourse with their wives or mates.

During my research, I discovered that a majority of men who suffer from premature ejaculation do not try to compensate for their sexual dysfunction. Some women married to premature ejaculators stated that their men do not even kiss them or caress them in any fashion. The majority of these men will not seek medical help and many of them are in denial and blame their mate for their sexual dysfunction.

I also discovered that those women who were in touch with their own sexuality were able to ask for what they wanted and needed sexually from their men in spite of their impotency and premature ejaculation. These women were much happier women. Those women who could not ask for what they wanted because of their fear of rejection and fear of hurting their partner's ego, felt angry, abused, frustrated and used- - - especially when their partner never discussed the dilemma by acting as though he though everything was alright. These women sometimes walked out of the relationship without giving any reason for doing so.

Chapter Eleven deals with the recipe for sexual fulfillment. This chapter will enlighten and enhance a man's knowledge and his ability to give much pleasure to his mate with or without an erected penis.

Many marriages have been broken up because of premature ejaculation. It is important for men and women to know that premature ejaculation can be cured. A couple must be willing to work together to make it a shared experience. As a result of this, the couple will grow closer together with a more enjoyable and gratifying sexual relationship, and the cure will be more effective. The "cure" occurs when the man can prevent himself from ejaculating until he and his partner are both satisfied, at least most of the time.

Men should not ignore sexual challenges. Sexual difficulty spills over into every aspect of one's life and activities. Next to eating, good sex is the next most sought after experience by humans.

A healthy energized body and mind can certainly enhance your sexual experience. Good nutrition and herbal products along with a good colon cleanser will help provide the body with the energy and vitality needed to improve one's overall well being- - - which can lead to a better sex life.

Chapter

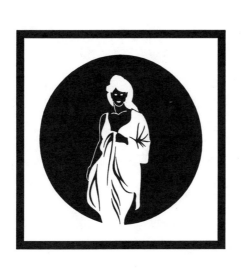

7

What Really Turns Her On

A diagram of the female external reproductive organs and vestibular bulbs.

This diagram is designed to give you a better insight as to what part of the female genitalia give the most pleasure when stimulated. The explanation of this diagram was taken from the Hite Report, which is a nationwide study of female sexuality.

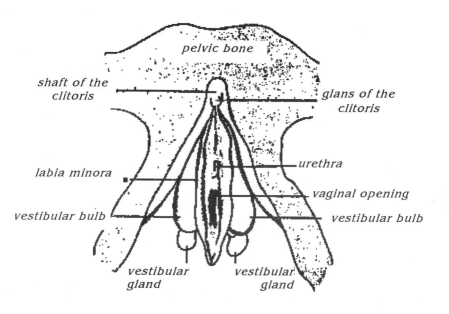

"The vestibular bulbs and the circum-vaginal plexus (a network of nerves, veins, and arteries) constitute the major erectile bodies in women. These underlying structures are homologous to, and about the same as, the penis of a man.

They become engorged (swollen) in the same way that a penis does. When fully engorged, the clitoral system as a whole is roughly thirty times as large as the external clitoral glans and shaft- - - what we commonly know as the clitoris.

Female sex organs, though internal and not as easily visible as men's, expand during arousal to approximately the same volume as an erected penis. The next time she is aroused notice how swollen [her] vulva and labia majora become; this reflects the swelling of the vestibular bulbs and other tissues, which lie just below this area.

In short, the only real difference between men's and women's erections is that men's are on the outside of their bodies, while women's are on the inside. Think of the clitoris as just the tip of you "penis," the rest of which lies underneath the surface of the vulva- - - or think of a penis as just the externalization of a women's interior bulbs and clitoral network.

The truth is…that the glans and shaft of the human clitoris are merely the superficially visible or palpable manifestations of an underlying clitoral system which is at least as large, as impressive, and as functionally responsive as the penis- - - and which responds as a unit sexual stimulation in much the same way that the penis does.

The penis, for example, has two roots known as crura which play an essential role in its functioning. During sexual excitation these crura become engorged with blood and contribute to erection of the penis. The clitoris, too, has two broad roots, of approximately the same size as in the male. The clitoral crura, too, become engorged with blood early in the woman's sexual excitation.

Again, the penis contains within its shaft two caverns or spaces known as corpora cavernosa, which fill with blood during sexual excitation, and contribute to the expanded size of the erect penis. The female clitoral system has a precisely analogous pair of bulbous corpora cavernosa, which similarly fill with blood during sexual excitation. They are not inside the shaft of the clitoris, however. Rather, they are located surrounding the vestibule and outer third of the vagina."

If this is new knowledge to you, please do not get excited and throw away all what you have been doing. I am sure that some of what you are doing is O.K. Do not be embarrassed if you have been going about it half right all these years. Remember, it is better to learn late than never.

Do not be embarrassed or ashamed to allow your woman to teach you how to bring her to an orgasm from clitoral stimulation. there are some things about a woman that a man will never know unless she tells him. For instance:

Whether she has had an orgasm or not.

Whether she is a virgin or not.

Whether she has had a hysterectomy or not.

Right now take the time to admit to yourself that you are a great lover realizing that no one knows it all and there is always room for improvement, more knowledge, and ultimately more sexual satisfaction. Now give her what she needs and has been wanting for a long time - - - an orgasm with intercourse. Remember, clitoral stimulation takes place externally and internally. Ask your woman for a little couching with your new ventures.

I will now discuss sexual responses gathered from a two- year survey of over 1,000 Black Women nationwide, professional and non-professional, between the ages of 19 to 75. The survey did not take into consideration origin of birth, religious preference, occupation, income level or martial status.

I realize that the above categories have a great influence on answers to the questions asked in the survey. However, a deeper and more precise study is in progress.

Each Time You Have Sex, Do You Have An Orgasm?

1% Said Yes
99% Said No

Does Your Sexual Partner Know When You Have Had An Orgasm?

60% Said Yes
15% Said No
25% Said Sometimes

Do You Fake Orgasm?

65% Said Yes
25% Said No
10% Said Sometimes

If You Fake Orgasm, Why?

"I want him to hurry up and get off me, and I

want to make him think he was satisfying me."

"Because I wanted my sex partner to feel that I could satisfy him."

"So as my partner will not be upset, because he did not fulfill my need."

"Because I did not want to deal with his anxieties if I didn't have one."

"So he can quit."

What Would You Like Your Sexual Partner To Do While You Are Experiencing An Orgasm?

"Relax."

"Foreplay."

"Whatever, I tell him to do."

"Kiss me."

"Have one at the same time."

"Talk to me."

"To rub my clitoris."

"Enjoy it with me, and if possible, enjoy one of his own."

"Continue to make love and talk to me."

"To relax and hold still because the ball is in my court."

"Touch me all over my body."

"Move with me and have an orgasm."

"Give all he's got."

"Continue what he was doing at the time of the orgasm - - make no changes, please.

"Have You Experienced Orgasm Without Sex?

"Yes, during foreplay with each other - - - also clitoral stimulation."

"Yes, by self- masturbation."

"I think so...in my dreams, however, I don't know if it's a physical orgasm or simply a mental one."

"Yes, by thinking of a sexual partner."

Do You Enjoy Clitoral Stimulation?

"Yes, if he is gentle."

95% Yes
4% No
1% Sometimes

Do You Like Your Sexual Partner To Express Himself Verbally During Sexual Intercourse?

"Yes, it makes me feel I am in control."

"Yes, to tell me what he likes."

(ALL THE WOMEN ANSWERED YES, EXCEPT THREE.)

What Words Do You Enjoy Hearing During Intercourse?

"None, really."

"I love you."

"I missed this good stuff."

"How great he feels."

"Hum...this is too good."

"My name."

"How good it is."

"Baby oh, give it to me."

"Baby, I'm coming."

"I feel good...you know the rest."

"Not too many vulgar words."

"Do you like it right here? Can you feel me? Want some more? I love you."

"I like to know how he's feeling. Talking dirty is fine as long as it is not vulgar."

"Oh, baby yes."

"How much he loves me...what a good partner I am."

Based on survey responses, many women like to hear their names called and to be reassured of their men's love for them during intercourse. My personal view is, a women should never fake an orgasm. Inflating a man's ego should never become a sexual liability for a woman. The energy spent, or shall I say wasted, on screaming, scratching, uttering untrue phrases, etc., could be utilized to focus on reaching total satisfaction for herself. I have been told by some men that what turns them on is `turning the woman on.' If this is true, faking an orgasm could drive him to a quicker climactic state in which he wins and the female faker loses.

Chapter

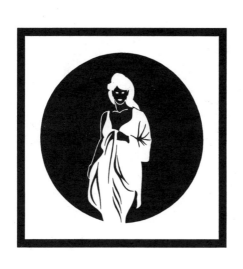

8

It is a known fact that many Black Women are single parents. Being single is a big problem within itself for some women- - - some but not all. Some single women view being single as a tragedy.

The fear of being alone is one of the greatest fears today among Black Women. The Black Woman is the woman most frequently left alone to rear her children. this fear is so overwhelming that it causes the black woman to fear communicating her sexual likes and dislikes.

The media's propaganda regarding the present and future outlook of the Black man is causing fear and excessive anxieties among Black Women. The Black man's future outlook tends to headline the major newspapers and is today's major discussion on television and talk shows where Blacks are being discussed. No other woman, other than the Black Woman is constantly reminded daily via print media and television that her man is an endangered species. Neither is there statistical information given regularly regarding how many men other than Black men are in jail, or how many are expected to spend some time in jail or will be on parole, etc.

The Black Woman is the most frequent victim of rape and assault today. The rape epidemic has become so widespread that one out of every three women in this country can expect to be raped at some point during her life. All women, not just "certain types" are potential rape victims; therefore, women live in fear of being raped, the Black Woman in particular.

Many women feel that being raped is their

fault. Because of the feelings of guilt and shame many women do not seek counseling. This leaves all the feelings kept inside of them hurting for a lifetime. Many times a woman will not discuss it with her partner because she fears how he may judge her as being the cause of the rape, instead of the victim. This is because many people in this society blame the woman who is raped. Men who do understand these dilemmas can clearly understand the reasons that many Black Women appear so strained.

Fears and anxieties greatly impact sexuality. All a Black woman will or will not do in bed or out of bed is a result of her "self image" derived from her total life experiences.   Angela Y. Davis, in her book, <u>Violence Against Women and The Ongoing Challenge to Racism</u>, included a portion of an article published in 1971 by Susan Griffin, a historic article in <u>Ramparts Magazine</u>, entitled "Rape: The All American Crime."

> "I have never been free of the fear of rape. From a very early age, I, like most women, have thought of rape as part of my natural environment- - - something to be feared and prayed against like fire or lightning. I never asked why men raped; I simply though it was one of the many mysteries of human nature.
>
> At the age of eight...my grandmother took me to the back of the house where the men wouldn't hear, and told me that strange men wanted to do harm to little girls. I learned not to walk on dark streets, not to talk to strangers or get into strange cars, to lock doors, and to be modest. She never explained why a man would want to harm a little girl, and I never asked.
>
> If I thought for a while that my grandmother's fears were imaginary, the illusion was brief. That year, on the way home from school, a schoolmate

a few years older than I, tried to rape me. Later, in an obscure aisle of the local library (while I was reading Freddy, the Pig), I turned to discover a man exposing himself. Then, the friendly man around the corner was arrested for child molesting."

Many Black Women experience much fear because of their lack of economic empowerment. The Black Woman continues to be the lowest paid in the employment sector. Merely providing the basic needs for her family becomes a constant challenge.

Many Black Women live in constant fear for the safety of their children because of the violence and crime which is at an all time high, especially in the inner city. Many fear their children may become involved in drug selling because of economic deprivation. Many Black Women find it very hard to be in a relaxed and peaceful state of mind, even in the arms of the man they desire being with so much, when their children are away from home at night.

Many Black Women are afraid to ask their men for any type of assistance or favors for fear that she will be labeled a "gold digger." During my research, I have not found that Black Women ask for any more material things than other women. If there is any truth in the stereotyping that the Black Woman asks for more, could it be that the Black Woman asks for more because she has less?

Below is a list of fears Black woman share:

"I may never get married unless I marry outside my race, because of the unavailability of Black men."

"If I go to bed with him, he will not marry me."

"If I do not go to bed with him, he will not marry me."

"If I say yes to sex too soon, he may think I am easy."

"If I divorce him, I may be single forever."

"If I do not make this marriage work, I may be viewed as a failure."

"If I divorce him, I will no longer be invited to social functions given by our old married friends."

"I fear not making it financially."

"I fear for my children safety."

"I fear my daughter may become pregnant."

"I fear aging,, because most men like young women."
"I fear that my man may try to seduce my daughter."

What Are Your Fears when Engaging In Sex With A Man To Whom You Are Not Married?

"Getting AIDS."

"Getting infections."

"Pregnancy and AIDS."

"Will he think less of me? Is this all he wants? The usual insecurities.."

"The wrath of God."

"Catching diseases if he is sleeping with someone else."
"My religious belief will haunt me."
"I have no fear because I will wait until I have known him for awhile before I have sex with him."

"V.D. and AIDS."

"Does he really care for me."

"Is this a one night affair or will he want more or what if I want more and he is out of my life."

"No fears because I believe in one partner."

"Past experiences and diseases."

"Getting AIDS etc. and don't forget the movie Fatal Attraction."

(Many mentioned AIDS and pregnancy.)

When Your Mate Is Having A Sexual Affair With Another Woman, Do You Think It Has

Something To Do With What You Are Doing Or Not Doing?

"Maybe."

"No. I just think he is a worthless ass."

"It is his life. He has the right to do this."

"I once felt that way but no more."

"Yes, but I am not willing to endanger my health by giving into his sexual exotic desires."

"It may and then again it may not."

"My man is not having any affairs outside of our relationship."

A vast majority of the women felt that if their man was having sex with another woman it had nothing to do with what they were doing or not doing.

Would You divorce Your Husband If He Is Sexually Involved With Another Woman?

"Probably. Since sex is not our problem I would have to think it was me."

"The answer is more complex than a mere yes or no - - - perhaps."

"I probably would because my ego would

be hurt."

"I might as well,, because I would never forgive him or trust him."

"Yes, because of AIDS."

"Yes, if other people know about it, especially my friends and family."

"That would certainly be my response but I would be willing (I think) to discuss it or seek counseling."

"Maybe not if this was the first time."

"No, if he does not continue it."

"It depends on whether or not he is a good provider."

"I experienced this early in my marriage. I am now married over 20 years- - - more mature with much more confidence in myself. If this should happen now no question- - - I would possible divorce.

More than 50 percent of the women said yes they would divorce their husband.

* *

Dear Men:

If you are married and your wife discovers that you are having an affair with another woman, the best you can do is be honest.

Do not try to blame your wife, please. What your wife needs from you is reassurance that you do not love her any less because you are involved with someone else.

Explain to her the real truth. If she chooses to end the relationship at least she can leave feeling good about herself. You should love her enough to care about her future.

Outside affairs make some relationships stronger while others fall apart. Remember, the risk begins the minute you get involved with another woman.

When your wife discovers that you have another woman, be prepared to make a choice. If you drag along trying to hold the girlfriend off until you decide what to do, you may soon discover that you have lost them both.

When women start battling over you, it is not about you. It is about their own ego of who wins.

A man or woman may find themselves attracted to another person. The reason for such is beyond the human understanding. It is something that sometimes happens. some people act on what they feel while others do not. Remember never to serve more than you can eat.

Sincerely yours,

Dr. Rosie Milligan

Would You Sever A Relationship With Your Mate If He Is Seeing Another Woman?

"Depends upon a lot of variables."

"Depends on the situation."

"In a courtship- - - Yes!"

More than 50 percent of the women said "yes."

"Maybe" and "no" answers were about equal.

Would You Date A Man Who Is Seeing Another Woman Already?

"Yes, if he is not my only man."

"Depending on circumstances- - - not an ongoing affair."

"Yes, if he is not living with her or married to her."

"All night long."

The majority of the women answered "no" to this question.

Would You Share Your Mate? If Yes, Describe Under What Circumstances?

"Not knowingly."

"Yes...with equal loving treatment from my ideal man, providing he told me about the other woman instead of my having to find out."

"Only if he is not my only man."

All other answers were "no," and "not knowingly."

Chapter

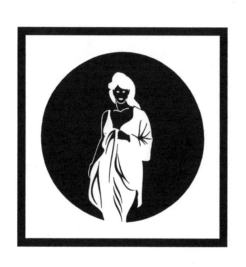

9

Women of all ethnic groups have identified some types of hang- ups. The hang- ups they all describe are directly related to their culture, history, personal and past experiences and family members past experiences. These are some of the hang- ups identified or shared by some Black Women.

* Feeling that her man does not love her if he has an affair with another woman.

* Judging her man on past experiences with other men in her past life.

* Never wanting to love again after being hurt.

* Afraid to become totally committed after a tragic relationship.

* Feeling guilty about entering a relationship shortly after the death of her husband.

* Feeling guilty or ashamed to marry a man her husband knew previously before his death or divorce.

* Believing the old quote, "Once a cheater, always a cheater."

Following are some of the responses gathered from a recent survey conducted on Black Women regarding sexual hang- ups.

Do You Have Any Sexual Hang-Ups? If So, Describe Them.

"Yes, I did not lose my virginity until I was 26 years old. As such, I feel less

knowledgeable about sex and sometimes feel less desirable. It also interferes with my ability to experience an orgasm sometimes."

"Yes...oral sex to me."

"Yes. I like foreplay before intercourse."

"Yes...but no anal sex for me."

"Sometimes I do not like for my breasts to be touched."

"Yes...feeling like I have to pretend I am enjoying sex when I am not."

"I hate clitoral stimulation during penile penetration."

"Yes. I do not like to have sex with the lights on."

A vast majority of the women said they had no sexual hang- ups.

Chapter

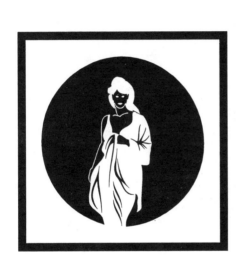

10

Times When A
Black Woman Does Not Want Sex

There are times when the Black Woman will not want sex. These are the times when her man should express understanding on the highest level. These are the times a woman appreciates love .... not sex.

* When she is on her menstrual cycle.

* When the children are awake and are up playing in the house.

* When death has occurred in the family.

* When the whereabouts of her child is unknown - (short term).

* When her child is in trouble - (remember, the Black Woman mother- child bonding).

* After an argument.

* When she is distressed financially.

* When her man has been unfaithful. (This holds true for a long time.)

Following are some of the responses from a recent survey conducted on Black Women regarding their sexual readiness.

Name The Times, Circumstances or Happenings When You Are Not Conducive to Good Sex - - -
(meaning when you cannot put your all into it).

"Tired physically or ill."

"When I have problems at work and at home."

"When my mind is filled with problems."

"If I am not feeling well, or if I do not feel clean."

"After a stressful day at the office."

"After a real heated argument."

"When I am mad at my mate."

"When preoccupied with more important matters."

"When my mind is other places."

"When I am awakened from my good sleep."

"When someone is up in the house walking around or when the children are not in bed asleep."

"When I am having financial problems."

How Do You Feel When You Have Had An Argument Or Have Been Provoked To Heated Anger And Your Mate Wants To Have Sex Before Resolving The Matter?

"I don't have sex with him until we have made up, and sometimes that takes a long time."

"Will not give in."

Used, angry, hurt and misunderstood."

"Depends, I may want to."

"I will not do it."

"I feel like killing the bastard."

"When the issue is not resolved, my mind will not be on sex. It makes me damn angry because he is the only one that benefits. He comes and I cannot. I consider this abuse."

"Like, stay away from me, because I do not want to be used."

"When we have had a fight or argument, we tend to make- up with sex. It's just one way of saying we are sorry and let's make- up."

"We will need to resolve any negative matters prior to lovemaking."

"Like an object."

"Disgusted."

"It angers me! Men can dismiss themselves from any situation to have sex. They (men) are so able to practice detachment."

"I usually make love and talk later. I do not believe in using sex as a weapon towards the other person."

"I don't."

"It doesn't happen- - - we resolve all

before we go to bed or we don't have sex. We never confuse the specialness of our love with Bullshit."

Wow! These answers were so emotionally charged, I said to myself, "I am glad I asked this question on paper and not in person!"

Chapter

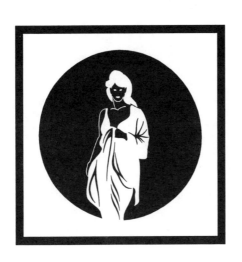

11

S atisfying the Black Woman sexually begins with making her feel special, loved, respected and cherished. Every woman wants to be pampered, adored and admired by her man every once and awhile. Men must realize that sex does not begin with stroking the body but begins with stroking the mind. Once she has the right mind set, her body will willingly follow. The key is to provide the right atmosphere so that her mind cannot help but be set on loving you totally and completely. Below are a few ingredients that should be added as often as necessary to savor, sweeten,, and spice up any relationship by creating an environment and mood more conducive for loving, sex and intimacy.

* *Be ever mindful as to where she has been and where she is presently.*

* *Be polite and kind.*

* *Remember sex and love making do not start in the bed. They start early in the morning when you pat her on the buttocks or just touch her nipples when she is stepping out of bed or when she is leaving the house. (This is like sauteing and flavoring a dish you want to cook when you get home.)*

* *When you hurt her, simply apologize instead of sending flowers.*

* *Send flowers spontaneously on non- special occasions.*

* *Call her at work just to say, "I love you."*

* *Call to let her know you cannot wait until she*

gets home. You may want to tease her by saying, "Honey, how long is it going to take you to get home" or "Can I meet you halfway, even better, sweetheart, let me pick you up from work - we can come back later for your car."

* Have soothing music playing when she comes home.

* Wear her favorite scented cologne, body lotion and aftershave lotion. Lay out that favorite lingerie you like seeing her wear.

* Prepare the bath water and make the bathroom cozy.

* Place a candle light in the bathroom and make scented bubble bath water.

* Take a bath or shower together. Apply deodorant under the armpits. do not apply aftershave lotion or cologne on the body. Remember cosmetics smell good but taste bitter. The scented bubble bath will leave your body smelling good. You may want to apply a sweet scented gel on your body and on her body. Make sure the scented gel is a fragrance she likes. (It comes in all fruit flavors.)

* Guide her to the bedroom that has been prepared for her. You are to be very busy all the way from the bathroom to the bedroom. Hopefully you can make it to the bedroom, you may get sidetracked by the commode in the bathroom, the face bowl in the bathroom, the hamper in the hallway, the chair or couch in the den, the wall in the hallway, the door to the bedroom, etc., etc., etc. If by chance you make it to the bed, then massage her body with oil. Beginning with the hand in a descending and organized fashion is very important.

* *Begin with her hands. This helps with the anticipation and relaxation process.*

* *Kiss her lightly over the eyelid.*

* *Pull her lip into your mouth softly, gliding your tongue from side to side on her lip.*

* *Seal your lips over her mouth and give a gentle puff of air.*

* *Massage the earlobes gently in a circular motion. Glide the tongue over the surface of the earlobe, softly sucking the earlobe in between a fixed number of glides. Then, blow small puffs of smoothing warm air over the wet surface of each earlobe.*

* *Give special attention to the nipples. The nipples should be handled with delicacy for good stimulation and excitation. If you are rough with the nipples, it will cause pain and pain will cause the muscles to contract. Remember, your sole objective is total relaxation. Now over the nipples, glide your tongue in a circular motion clockwise then counter clockwise. Then, with medium pressure, blow warm air over the wet surface of the nipples.*

* *If the breast are large, pull the nipples close together and caress both at the same time. If the breasts are small, go from one to the other stimulating interchangeably in a circular motion with light pressure. Remember, the size of the breasts is not an issue.*

* *When you hit the hot button, you will notice a drastic change in her breathing pattern. Move away from the hot spot and search for other areas to explore. Every now and then come*

back to the hot button for another burst of pleasure.

* Before massaging the feet, apply a generous amount of oil over the palms of your hands. Start at the tip of the toes and work towards the heel. This usually relaxes the whole body.

* Massage the legs with light strokes proceeding in an upward and downward motion, moving from ankle to knee and from knee to ankle. Massage the thigh lightly with circular and crossing strokes.

* Lightly massage the belly button. Gently massage the pubic area with one hand while the other hand is massaging the nipples of the breast.

Very gently lubricate the clitoral and vaginal areas with Vaseline or KY jelly, etc. Glide your finger over the glans of the clitoris. Place your thumb and first finger over the glans of the clitoris. Very, very softly, open and close your fingers. Remember always to be tender but yet, sensitive to her responses, including increasing and decreasing in the frequency and intensity of the stimulation of various areas according to her body language, expressions and vocal gestures.

* If she has not raped you by now, then turn her over face down and massage her shoulders, back, buttocks and back of her legs. Remember every now and then, blow a warm breath of air over her body.

* Now give her a long good juicy kiss in the mouth and say to your woman, "Tell me when you are ready for me. Tell me how and where." Never assume the bed is the right place. There

should be times when you call the shots as related to positions and place. There should be times when your woman does the same.

* *Take your woman or wife to a hotel sometimes. Welcome new ideas from your woman or wife. A woman often likes romance without sex. When single, take your woman out for fun without sex. It will heighten her desire for you the next time around.*

* *Often a woman's job can be quite challenging, especially when she is in management. Be prepared to make her smile when she comes home instead of waiting for her to always make your day. If you follow these simple steps and use the aforementioned ingredients, you will be happy - morning, noon, and night. Love never grows old; it ages like wine and becomes stronger. Always remember...when you are busy spreading sunshine, the sun has to shine on you.*

Let's look at a few simple things that can add spice to life. Write your woman love notes. Send her your love notes, friendship, and thinking of you cards through the mail. Leave a note on her pillow describing how you plan to make love to her when you come home, or a note telling her how much you enjoyed her last night, etc. Once in a while, go to her job or place of business and leave a miscellaneous note in her car, attached to the steering wheel. On the note, describe what you have waiting for her if she gets home by a designated time. Lounge around the house in your robe with nothing on under it. While kissing your woman, open your robe and wrap it around her.

The following items are samples

of a communique that you can

send to your woman for fun

Prescription

Name _____ Date _____

Address _____

RX Massage to be given by _____
who will apply exotic Love Gel or stimulating lotion to your
entire body _____

To be Refilled _____ Times

Signed _____
Your Personal Love Doctor

Address _____ Phone _____

Prescription Certificate

Name _____ Date _____

Address _____

Rx

☐ Dispense as written ☐ Substitutions permitted ☐ Refillable ___ (times)

Dr _____
    Your Personal Care Doctor

Address _____ Phone _____

Massage Messenger

This Certificate Entitles : _____

To the following services : _____

Performed by: _____

Expiration Date: _____

Telephone Sex

If your woman is long distance, an orgasm is just a phone call away. You can make love to your woman via telephone. Making love via telephone can be a gratifying experience. the phone method allows one to be very creative, uninhibited, and talkative. It really allows one to share experiences that one could not share comfortably in person.

Ask your woman what she is wearing? Then tell her step by step how to take off each piece, (e.g., take off your dress and lay it aside; take off your bra and lay it aside; take off your shoes and stockings; get in the bed and lie on your back). Then ask if she is wearing panties. If yes, say to her, "Sweetheart, lift up your buttocks and slide them off." Remember, the bed is not always the place; therefore, you create the scene according to your mood and sexual appetite. You explain explicitly, detailed and erotically everything you are doing to her. Since you cannot see the expression of your woman; tell her that she needs to verbally tell you what she is feeling. You will find yourself doing and saying things that you may not feel comfortable doing or saying in person. If your woman has sexual toys, guide her step by step as to what she is to be doing with them. Ask her to let you know what she feels. if she wants you to do something different than what you are describing to her, in order to give her more pleasure, you are to adhere to her request and verbally tell her erotically what you are doing to her and for her.

If your woman is not long distance and you

want to have this experience, go into a different room in the house and have her pick up the phone. Just pretend that it is long distance. Making love on the phone can be good and safe.

As an added "dish" to the recipe for sexual fulfillment, you may consider using herbs. For better energy and stamina, consider the herbal approach. Herbs can enhance the sexuality for you and your partner.

The following is a list of herbs and what they are used for:

Sexual Impotency and Sexual Stimulant

Ginseng
Damiana
Formula I Juice
STIF Herbal Tonic

Vitality and Energy

CKLS
Ginseng
Bee Pollen
Formula I Juice
Gota Kola
Royal Jelly

Colon Cleanser

CKLS
Pure Olive Oil
Cascara Sagrada
LBS

Prostate

CKLS
Zinc
Uva Ursi

Anemia

4- PG
Dandelion
Yellow Dock

High Blood Pressure

BP- 1
BP- 2
Garlic

Weight Loss

Par- K Slim Pack
Chickweed

Brain Booster

CKLS
Gota Kola
Fo Ti Tieng

Circulation

Capsicum
Formula I Juice

NOTE: If after reading this book you find you are in need of sex counseling, call Professional Business Consulting Service for a referral source at the number below.

PROFESSIONAL BUSINESS CONSULTING SERVICES

(213) 750- 3592

or

Visit our Health Food Store at:

2108 W. Manchester Ave.
Los Angeles, Ca. 90047

(213) 751- 3214

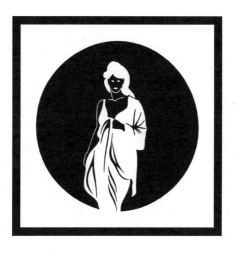

We have travelled a Great distance since the beginning of this book. I certainly hope you enjoyed the journey. More importantly, I sincerely hope that you and your partner will benefit from the thoughts shared here, for that was my ultimate goal.

I, like most of us, have seen many relationships destroyed by misunderstandings in the sexual area. This need not be the case. If the tecniques and ideas imparted here are adapted to your situation, I am convinced it will make a positive difference. Try it. Simply do s- o- m- e- t- h- i- n- g from this book today, right now if possible. Don't be afraid. If your partner asks where you learned that, show him the book.

And don't feel that you need to copy the ideas verbatim, use them to stimulate your own creative Juices. If you think of something new, do it! Remember, two consenting adults can do anything they desire in private. Too often we stifle ourselves. If you do, take action to stop.

Be kind to our Black women whenever possible. They deserve it. They have a dubious distinction in America. If anyone deserves a break, they do. Please don't misunderstand me, everyone should be treated with kindness, you included.

If that has not been the case in your relationship, I suggest you start the ball rolling. Someone has to begin.

I feel like I just heard a collective groan from Black Men throughout the United States that sounded like:

"Why do I have to be the one? Why can't She go first for a change?" The answer is simple, if she hasn't in the past, it is highly unlikely that she will in the future without a different motivation.

You can provide that motivation. Few people will take and take and take. If you give more, you will usually get more in return. Try it. You have very little to lose and a lot to gain!!

Good luck and may God bless you.

Reference Books
....

1) *Medical Aspects of Human Sexuality*
   Special Issue - The Physician 's Guide to the Management
   of Impotence .. April 1989

2) Brothers, Joyce, Dr.
   What Every Woman Should Know About Men
   Ballantine Books, New York

3) Williams & Wilkins
   Baltimore - London - Los Angeles - Sydney
   Understanding Human Behavior in Health and Illness
   Third Edition ... Edited by Richard C. Simons, M.D.

4) Zilbergeld, Bernie, Ph.D.
   The New Male Sexuality
   Bantam Books, New York

5) Madhubuti, Haki R.
   Obsolete, Single, Dangerous?
   Third World Press, 1990

6) Barashango, Ishakamusa, Rev. D.
   Afrikan Woman The Original Guardian Angel
   IVth Dynasty Publishing Company, 1989

7) Welsing, Cress Frances, M.D.
   The Isis (Yssis) Papers
   Third World Press

8) *"J" The Sensuous Woman*
   Dell Publishing Company, 1982

9) Hite Shere
   The Hits Report
   Dell Publishing Company, 1976

10) Schwartz, Bob
    One Hour Orgasm
    Breakthru Publishing, 1988

11) Kennedy, Adele P. and Dean, Susan. Ph.D.
Touching for Pleasure
Chatsworth Press. 1986

12) Davis, Angela Y.
Violence Against Women and the Ongoing Challenge to Racism
Women of Color Press, 1985

13) Berkeley Holistic Health Center
The Holistic Health Handbook,
And/Or Press, 1978

14) Hooks, Bell
Ain't I A Woman
South End Press, 1981

15) Sims, Claudette Elaine
Don't Weep For Me
Impressions

16) Rodgers-Rose, La Frances
The Black Woman
Sage Publications

Suggested Reading

Giddings, Paula
When and Where I Enter
Bantam. Books

Scott, Kesho Yvonne
The Habit of Surviving
Rutgers University Press

King, Victoria
Manhandled Black Females
Winston-Derek, Nashville, Tennessee

BOOKS AVAILABLE THROUGH
Professional Business Consultants
by Dr. Rosie Milligan

Satisfying the Blackwoman Sexually Made Simple -$14.95
Satisfying the Blackman Sexually Made Simple -$14.95
Negroes-Colored People-Blacks-African-Americans in America- $13.95
Starting A Business Made Simple - $20.00
Getting Out of Debt Made Simple - $20.00

-------------------------------Order Form-------------------------------

Mail Check or Money Order to: 2108 W. Manchester, Suite C, Los Angeles, CA 90047

Name_____Date_____

Address_____

City_____ State _____ Zip Code _____

Day Telephone _____

Eve Telephone _____

Name of book(s) _____

Sub Total $_____

Sales Tax (CA Add 8.25%) $_____

Shipping & Handling $3.00 $_____

Total Amount Due $_____

☐ Check   ☐ Money Order

☐ Visa   ☐ Master Card   Ex. Date _____

Credit Card No. _____

Driver's License No._____

_____   _____

Signature   Date

NOTES

NOTES

NOTES

NOTES